Unleashing the Warrior Within: A Journey through the Martial Arts World

"U"nleashing the Warrior Within: A Journey through the Martial Arts World" is a captivating exploration of the multifaceted world of martial arts. From the ancient traditions of Asia to the modern combat disciplines practiced worldwide, this book takes readers on an immersive journey that delves into the history, philosophy, techniques, and transformative power of martial arts. It offers a unique blend of storytelling, personal experiences, and expert insights, providing a comprehensive guide for both martial arts enthusiasts and those curious to learn more.

Embark on a quest to discover the essence of martial arts —the deep-rooted traditions, the physical prowess, the mental fortitude, and the spiritual growth that come with the practice. Explore the diverse range of martial arts styles, from the striking arts like Karate, Taekwondo, and Muay Thai, to the grappling arts like Brazilian Jiu-Jitsu and Judo. Uncover the secrets of ancient disciplines such as Kung Fu and Aikido, and learn about the modern self-defense systems like Krav Maga and Jeet Kune Do.

But "Unleashing the Warrior Within" is more than just a catalog of martial arts styles. It delves into the underlying philosophies and principles that shape these arts, such as discipline, respect, perseverance, and humility. It delves into the mental and emotional aspects of martial arts training, exploring the benefits of increased self-confidence, stress relief, and personal growth.

Through captivating narratives, the book shares the stories of legendary martial artists who have left an indelible mark on the world. From Bruce Lee's revolutionary philosophy to the indomitable spirit of Mas Oyama, their journeys serve as inspiration for all those who seek to embark on their own martial arts path.

Moreover, "Unleashing the Warrior Within" highlights the broader cultural and historical significance of martial arts. It explores the role of martial arts in ancient warfare, the evolution of martial arts in different regions, and the impact of martial arts on popular culture, including movies and martial arts tournaments.

Whether you are an aspiring martial artist, a seasoned practitioner, or someone intrigued by the world of martial arts, this book will captivate your imagination and deepen your understanding. "Unleashing the Warrior Within: A Journey through the Martial Arts World" is a guide that invites you to embrace the physical and mental challenges, uncover your inner strength, and embark on a transformative journey of self-discovery.

Introduction

- The power and allure of martial arts
- Purpose and Scope of the book

Chapter 1: The Origins of Martial Arts

- Ancient martial arts in China, Japan, and other regions

- Mental and emotional benefits of martial arts training
- Building self-confidence and self-awareness
- Stress relief and mental well-being
- Balancing physical and mental development

Chapter 7: Martial Arts in Culture and Society

- Martial arts in warfare and self-defense throughout history
- Influence of martial arts on popular culture and media
- Martial arts tournaments and their impact

Chapter 8: Embarking on Your Martial Arts Journey

- Choosing the right martial art for you
- Finding the right instructor and training environment
- Setting goals and tracking progress
- Overcoming challenges and staying motivated

Conclusion

- Reflection on the transformative power of martial arts
- Final thoughts and encouragement for readers
- Resources for further exploration

The power and allure of martial arts

The power and allure of martial arts are undeniable. It is a discipline that has fascinated people for centuries, captivating both participants and observers with its dynamic movements, ancient traditions, and profound philosophies. From the graceful strikes of a masterful kick to the intense grappling techniques of a seasoned practitioner, martial arts possess a unique ability to captivate and inspire.

At its core, martial arts is more than just a physical practice—it is a way of life. The power of martial arts lies in its ability to transform individuals, not only physically but also mentally and emotionally. It teaches discipline, resilience, and perseverance, instilling a strong work ethic and a never-give-up attitude. Through rigorous training, martial artists develop strength, speed, agility, and endurance, pushing their bodies to new limits.

However, martial arts is not solely about physical prowess. It delves deep into the realm of the mind and spirit. The allure of martial arts lies in the philosophical and spiritual principles it embraces. Concepts such as respect, humility, and self-control are at the core of martial arts philosophy, guiding practitioners to cultivate inner peace and harmony.

The practice of martial arts also offers a pathway for self-discovery and personal growth. It challenges individuals to confront their fears and limitations, pushing them to become the best versions of themselves. Through the demanding physical training and mental focus required, martial arts practitioners gain a heightened sense of self-awareness and learn to harness their inner strength.

Beyond the individual benefits, martial arts has the power to foster a sense of community and connection. Martial arts schools and dojos often become spaces where like-minded individuals come together, supporting and inspiring one another on their martial arts journeys. This sense of camaraderie and mutual respect extends beyond the training mat, creating lifelong friendships and a global network of martial arts enthusiasts.

Moreover, martial arts carries with it a rich cultural heritage and history. Each style of martial art is deeply rooted in its cultural origins, reflecting the values, traditions, and rituals of its respective region. The allure of martial arts lies not only in the physical movements but also in the connection to these ancient lineages and the preservation of cultural heritage.

Whether practiced for self-defense, fitness, competition, or personal growth, martial arts has an undeniable power to captivate and inspire. Its allure lies in its ability to simultaneously challenge and uplift individuals, allowing them to tap into their inner warrior and unleash their full potential. The power of martial arts goes beyond the physical—it reaches deep into the soul, shaping character, and transforming lives.

Purpose and Scope of the book

The purpose of "Unleashing the Warrior Within: A Journey through the Martial Arts World" is to provide a comprehensive exploration of the multifaceted world of martial arts. The book aims to educate and inspire readers by delving into the history, philosophy, techniques, and transformative power of martial arts.

The scope of the book encompasses a wide range of topics related to martial arts. It covers the origins of martial arts, tracing its roots back to ancient civilizations and highlighting its evolution over time. It explores different martial arts styles, including striking arts, grappling arts, traditional forms, and modern self-defense systems. The book delves into the philosophy and principles underlying martial arts, emphasizing concepts such as discipline, respect, and mental fortitude.

The training and techniques section provides insights into fundamental movements, striking and grappling techniques, forms, and sparring. It also explores the mental and emotional aspects of martial arts training, highlighting the benefits of increased self-confidence, stress relief, and personal growth.

Additionally, the book offers profiles and stories of legendary martial artists who have made significant contributions to the field. It examines their philosophies, experiences, and legacies, providing inspiration and lessons that readers can apply to their own martial arts journeys.

The book goes beyond the physical aspects of martial arts by exploring its broader cultural and historical significance. It discusses the role of martial arts in warfare, its influence on popular culture, and the impact of martial arts tournaments.

"Unleashing the Warrior Within" aims to be a valuable resource for both martial arts enthusiasts and individuals who are curious about the world of martial arts. It seeks to provide a comprehensive guide that covers various aspects of martial arts, allowing readers to deepen their understanding, gain practical insights, and find inspiration for their own martial arts journeys.

Ancient martial arts in China, Japan, and other regions

Ancient martial arts in China, Japan, and other regions hold a significant place in the history and development of martial arts as we know them today. These ancient practices were deeply rooted in the cultures and traditions of their respective regions, and their influence continues to be felt in modern martial arts disciplines.

In China, the origins of martial arts can be traced back thousands of years. Ancient Chinese martial arts, known as wushu or kung fu, encompassed a wide range of styles and techniques. These arts were developed as a means of self-defense and military training, with some styles originating from ancient battlefield tactics. Shaolin Temple, renowned for its role in the development and preservation of martial arts, is a symbol of Chinese martial arts' ancient roots.

Chinese martial arts emphasized both external and internal training. External training focused on physical conditioning, including strength, flexibility, and striking techniques. Internal training emphasized cultivating the mind, energy flow (qi or chi), and mastering internal martial arts principles such as Tai Chi and Bagua Zhang.

In Japan, ancient martial arts were deeply intertwined with the samurai warrior class and the code of bushido. The samurai practiced martial arts not only for self-defense but also as a means of personal development and spiritual growth. Japanese martial arts, such as Judo, Aikido, Karate, Kendo, and Kenjutsu, emerged from these ancient traditions.

Judo, created by Jigoro Kano in the late 19th century, was derived from the ancient grappling art of Jujutsu. Aikido, founded by Morihei Ueshiba, blended martial arts techniques with spiritual principles. Karate developed from Okinawan and Chinese influences and focused on striking techniques. Kendo, the way of the sword, preserved the techniques and philosophy of the samurai's swordsmanship.

In addition to China and Japan, other regions around the world also had their own ancient martial arts practices. For example, Southeast Asia has a rich history of martial arts, such as Muay Thai in Thailand, Silat in Indonesia, and Arnis/Eskrima in the Philippines. These arts were often deeply connected to cultural traditions, regional conflicts, and tribal practices.

The ancient martial arts in these regions not only served as practical combat systems but also played significant roles in shaping their respective cultures, values, and philosophies. They were passed down through generations, often within family lineages or secret societies, and preserved through oral tradition and practical application.

Studying the ancient martial arts in China, Japan, and other regions provides valuable insights into the historical, cultural, and philosophical foundations of martial arts. It allows practitioners to appreciate the depth of these arts and understand how they have evolved and influenced modern martial arts practices. Furthermore, exploring these ancient roots can deepen one's connection to the traditions and values that have been passed down through centuries of practice.

Influence of philosophy and spirituality

The influence of philosophy and spirituality in martial arts is profound and pervasive. Across different cultures and regions, martial arts have been deeply intertwined with philosophical and spiritual teachings, enhancing not only physical combat skills but also the development of one's character, mindset, and inner harmony.

One of the most well-known philosophical influences in martial arts is the concept of Zen Buddhism, particularly in Japanese martial arts. Zen emphasizes mindfulness, presence, and the cultivation of a clear and focused mind. It encourages practitioners to be fully present in each moment and to let go of distracting thoughts and emotions. This mindset is highly applicable in martial arts, where a calm and focused state of mind is essential for optimal performance and effective decision-making.

Another influential philosophy in martial arts is Taoism, originating from China. Taoism emphasizes the harmony and balance of opposites, represented by the concepts of yin and yang. In martial arts, this philosophy is often reflected in the concept of softness overcoming hardness, using an opponent's energy against them, and seeking balance and fluidity in movement. The principles of Taoism encourage martial artists to flow with the natural rhythms of the universe and to adapt to changing circumstances.

Spirituality is also an integral part of martial arts practice for many individuals. Some martial arts styles incorporate elements of meditation, breath control, and visualization techniques to cultivate a deeper connection with the self and the universe. This spiritual aspect helps practitioners develop self-awareness, discipline, and a sense of purpose beyond physical combat.

Martial arts also emphasize the cultivation of virtues such as respect, discipline, humility, and perseverance. These values are deeply rooted in the philosophical and spiritual foundations of the arts. Practitioners are encouraged to carry these principles beyond the training mat and into their daily lives, fostering personal growth, ethical conduct, and a positive impact on society.

Furthermore, the philosophical and spiritual aspects of martial arts provide a means for practitioners to explore their own sense of identity, purpose, and self-discovery. The journey of martial arts goes beyond mere physical techniques, as practitioners are encouraged to explore their strengths and weaknesses, confront their fears and limitations, and strive for personal growth and transformation.

By incorporating philosophy and spirituality, martial arts becomes a holistic discipline that encompasses not only physical training but also mental and spiritual development. It offers practitioners a pathway to self-improvement, self-discovery, and a deeper understanding of themselves and the world around them. The influence of philosophy and spirituality in martial arts enriches the practice, elevating it beyond mere combat skills and instilling a profound sense of purpose, mindfulness, and personal fulfillment.

Evolution of martial arts through history

The evolution of martial arts through history is a fascinating journey that spans centuries and encompasses a wide range of cultural, historical, and technological developments. From the ancient battlefield techniques of early civilizations to the modern martial arts disciplines practiced today, martial arts have continuously evolved and adapted to meet the changing needs and contexts of different times.

1. Ancient Origins:
    - The earliest evidence of martial arts can be traced back to ancient civilizations such as Mesopotamia, Egypt, and China. These early practices were primarily focused on combat skills for warfare and self-defense.
    - Ancient civilizations developed unique fighting systems, including hand-to-hand combat, weapons training, and military strategies. Examples include the Chinese art of Wushu, the Greek Pankration, and the Roman gladiatorial combat.
2. Asian Martial Arts:
    - In Asia, martial arts evolved alongside the growth of various civilizations and cultural exchanges.
    - In China, arts such as Kung Fu, Tai Chi, and Wing Chun emerged from the influence of Buddhist and Taoist philosophies, incorporating concepts of balance, energy flow, and spiritual development.

- In Japan, martial arts like Jujutsu, Kenjutsu, and Aikido were developed by samurai warriors, emphasizing disciplined techniques, honor, and bushido (the way of the warrior).

3. Codification and Modernization:
   - In the late 19th and early 20th centuries, martial arts underwent significant changes due to social and political shifts.
   - In Japan, Jigoro Kano developed Judo, focusing on safe and effective training methods and competitive sport elements. Gichin Funakoshi introduced Karate to mainland Japan from Okinawa, popularizing it as a modern martial art.
   - In China, martial arts were systematized into styles such as Shaolin Kung Fu and Tai Chi, making them more accessible to a broader audience.

4. Globalization and Hybridization:
   - With increased globalization and cultural exchange, martial arts spread beyond their countries of origin.
   - The introduction of martial arts to the West, through figures like Bruce Lee and his Jeet Kune Do philosophy, influenced the development of hybrid styles and cross-training methodologies.
   - The rise of mixed martial arts (MMA) in the late 20th century further showcased the effectiveness of blending different martial arts disciplines, leading to the development of MMA-specific training methods.

5. Contemporary Martial Arts:
   - Modern martial arts encompass a wide range of styles, each with its unique techniques, training methods, and philosophies.

- Martial arts continue to evolve, incorporating elements of sports science, strength and conditioning, and advancements in training equipment and technology.
- While some martial arts retain their traditional forms, others have adapted to contemporary contexts, such as Krav Maga for self-defense or Brazilian Jiu-Jitsu for sport grappling.

The evolution of martial arts through history reflects the influences of culture, philosophy, technological advancements, and societal changes. Today, martial arts continue to thrive, appealing to practitioners seeking self-defense skills, physical fitness, personal development, and cultural exploration. The rich and diverse history of martial arts serves as a testament to their enduring appeal and ongoing evolution.

Striking arts: Karate, Taekwondo, Muay Thai, etc.

Striking arts are a prominent category within the world of martial arts. These disciplines focus on the effective use of striking techniques, including punches, kicks, knees, and elbows. Here are a few notable striking arts:

1. Karate:
   - Originating in Okinawa, Japan, Karate is known for its powerful strikes and linear movements. It emphasizes proper form, precise timing, and breath control.
   - Karate training involves a combination of strikes, blocks, kicks, and stances. It promotes discipline, focus, and self-defense skills.
   - Karate has different styles, including Shotokan, Goju-Ryu, Wado-Ryu, and Kyokushin.

2. Taekwondo:
   - Developed in Korea, Taekwondo is renowned for its dynamic and high-flying kicks. It emphasizes speed, agility, and flexibility.
   - Taekwondo training involves a wide range of kicks, strikes, blocks, and acrobatic movements. It incorporates sparring, forms (poomsae), and breaking techniques.
   - Taekwondo is known for its competitive aspect and is an Olympic sport.

3. Muay Thai:
   - Originating in Thailand, Muay Thai is often

referred to as "The Art of Eight Limbs" because it utilizes punches, kicks, knees, and elbows.

- Muay Thai focuses on aggressive and powerful striking techniques, clinch work, and devastating knee and elbow strikes.
- Training in Muay Thai involves conditioning, pad work, sparring, and clinch drills. It is renowned for its effectiveness in combat sports and self-defense.

4. Boxing:

- Boxing is a Western combat sport that primarily focuses on punches and footwork. It emphasizes speed, accuracy, and defensive techniques.
- Boxing training involves shadowboxing, bag work, pad work, and sparring. It develops endurance, coordination, and timing.
- Boxing is an Olympic sport and a popular discipline for fitness and self-defense.

5. Kickboxing:

- Kickboxing combines elements of boxing and various kicking techniques from martial arts such as Karate, Taekwondo, and Muay Thai.
- Kickboxing training involves striking drills, pad work, bag work, and sparring. It develops cardiovascular fitness, strength, and striking proficiency.
- Kickboxing has different styles, including American Kickboxing, Dutch Kickboxing, and Full Contact Karate.

These striking arts offer unique training methods, techniques, and philosophies. While they may have originated from different regions and cultures, they share a common focus on developing effective striking skills, physical conditioning, and mental discipline. Whether practiced for self-defense, sport, fitness, or personal growth, striking arts provide practitioners with a platform to enhance their striking abilities, boost confidence, and cultivate discipline.

Grappling arts: Brazilian Jiu-Jitsu, Judo, Wrestling, etc.

Grappling arts are martial arts disciplines that emphasize controlling and subduing opponents through techniques such as throws, takedowns, joint locks, and chokeholds. These arts focus on close-range combat, ground fighting, and the application of leverage and technique. Here are a few notable grappling arts:

1. Brazilian Jiu-Jitsu (BJJ):
    - Developed in Brazil, BJJ is known for its effectiveness in ground fighting and submission holds. It emphasizes technique and leverage to overcome size and strength.
    - BJJ training focuses on grappling, positional control, and submissions. It includes techniques such as sweeps, joint locks, and chokes.
    - BJJ is popular in mixed martial arts (MMA) and submission grappling tournaments, where it has proven to be highly effective.

2. Judo:
    - Originating in Japan, Judo translates to "the gentle way." It emphasizes throwing and grappling techniques to overcome opponents.
    - Judo training includes learning how to off-balance opponents and execute precise throws. It also incorporates ground fighting techniques and submissions.
    - Judo is an Olympic sport and is known for

"

its emphasis on discipline, respect, and mutual welfare.

3. Wrestling:
   - Wrestling is a combat sport practiced in various forms across different cultures, including folkstyle, freestyle, and Greco-Roman.
   - Wrestling focuses on takedowns, throws, and controlling an opponent's body. It emphasizes strength, agility, and technique.
   - Wrestling is an Olympic sport and has been adapted into different styles, such as collegiate wrestling in the United States.

4. Sambo:
   - Sambo, originating in Russia, is a combination of wrestling, judo, and striking techniques. It was developed for both self-defense and combat sports.
   - Sambo training includes throws, takedowns, joint locks, and ground fighting techniques. It incorporates both standing and ground-based strategies.
   - Sambo is practiced in various forms, including Sport Sambo (competition) and Combat Sambo (military and self-defense application).

5. Catch Wrestling:
   - Catch Wrestling, originating in England, is a grappling style that combines techniques from various grappling arts.
   - Catch Wrestling emphasizes submissions, joint locks, and pinning techniques. It is known for its practicality and effectiveness in real-world combat.
   - Catch Wrestling has influenced modern grappling arts such as BJJ and submission grappling.

These grappling arts offer unique training methodologies, strategies, and techniques. While they have their specific origins and cultural influences, they all share a common emphasis on grappling, control, and submission techniques. Practicing grappling arts provides practitioners with a practical understanding of close-quarter combat, body mechanics, and leverage. Whether practiced for sport, self-defense, or personal growth, grappling arts offer a dynamic and challenging avenue for physical development, mental discipline, and strategic problem-solving.

Traditional and weapon-based arts: Kung Fu, Aikido, etc.

Traditional and weapon-based arts encompass martial arts disciplines that focus on traditional techniques, forms, and weapons. These arts often carry deep historical and cultural significance and emphasize the development of discipline, technique, and mastery. Here are a few notable traditional and weapon-based arts:

1. Kung Fu (Wushu):
    - Kung Fu, originating in China, encompasses a vast array of martial arts styles. It emphasizes fluidity, agility, and a combination of strikes, kicks, and grappling techniques.
    - Kung Fu training includes forms (katas), sparring, self-defense applications, and weapon training (such as the staff, sword, and nunchaku).
    - Kung Fu styles include Shaolin Kung Fu, Wing Chun, Tai Chi, and many others, each with its own unique techniques, philosophies, and training methods.

2. Aikido:
    - Aikido, developed in Japan, emphasizes using an opponent's energy and movements against them. It focuses on joint locks, throws, and redirection of force.
    - Aikido training includes techniques for both unarmed and armed attacks. It incorporates

circular movements, blending with the opponent's energy, and maintaining a centered and relaxed state.

- Aikido emphasizes harmony, non-aggression, and resolving conflicts without causing harm.

3. Kendo:

- Kendo, also known as the "Way of the Sword," is a Japanese martial art that focuses on swordsmanship.
- Kendo training involves using a bamboo sword (shinai) and protective armor (bogu). It emphasizes proper form, timing, and spirit in strikes, footwork, and defensive techniques.
- Kendo places a strong emphasis on discipline, respect, and the development of mental focus and awareness.

4. Eskrima/Arnis/Kali:

- Eskrima, Arnis, and Kali are Filipino martial arts that emphasize weapon-based techniques, primarily using sticks (escrima) or blades (arnis/kali).
- Eskrima training includes both empty-hand techniques and weapon techniques. It focuses on coordination, agility, and efficient use of weapons for self-defense.
- Eskrima/Arnis/Kali incorporates a range of techniques, including strikes, blocks, disarms, and grappling.

5. Kyudo:

- Kyudo, the Japanese martial art of archery, is known for its emphasis on form, precision, and meditation.
- Kyudo training involves shooting arrows from a traditional longbow (yumi) and focuses on the development of concentration, discipline, and proper breathing techniques.

- Kyudo places a strong emphasis on the connection between the archer's mind, body, and spirit.

These traditional and weapon-based arts offer practitioners an opportunity to connect with rich cultural traditions, develop discipline, and explore the intricacies of weaponry. Whether practicing empty-hand techniques or mastering weapon skills, these arts provide a unique approach to self-defense, personal growth, and historical preservation.

Modern self-defense systems: Krav Maga, Jeet Kune Do, etc.

Modern self-defense systems are martial arts disciplines that have been developed with a primary focus on practicality, efficiency, and real-world self-defense scenarios. These systems often borrow techniques from various martial arts and adapt them for real-life confrontations. Here are a few notable modern self-defense systems:

1. Krav Maga:
    - Krav Maga is a self-defense system developed in Israel, originally for the Israeli military. It emphasizes instinctive movements, practical techniques, and aggressive counterattacks.
    - Krav Maga training includes strikes, kicks, grappling, and defenses against common street attacks. It also incorporates training for multiple attackers, weapons defenses, and situational awareness.
    - Krav Maga's emphasis is on neutralizing threats quickly and efficiently, making it popular among law enforcement, military personnel, and civilians seeking practical self-defense skills.
2. Jeet Kune Do:
    - Jeet Kune Do (JKD), developed by Bruce Lee, is a philosophy and martial art that emphasizes simplicity, efficiency, and adapting to the situation.

- JKD incorporates techniques from various martial arts, including Boxing, Wing Chun, Fencing, and Filipino Martial Arts. It focuses on intercepting attacks, fluidity of movement, and economy of motion.
- JKD training includes striking, trapping, grappling, and weapons training. It encourages personal expression and the exploration of individual strengths and attributes.

3. Systema:

- Systema is a Russian martial art that focuses on developing natural movement, adaptability, and control of both oneself and the opponent.
- Systema training includes strikes, joint locks, and throws, as well as breath control, relaxation, and psychological preparation. It emphasizes efficient use of body mechanics and developing resilience in high-stress situations.
- Systema incorporates both unarmed and armed self-defense techniques and is known for its emphasis on continuous movement, fluidity, and relaxation under duress.

4. Defendo:

- Defendo is a Canadian self-defense system developed by Bill Underwood. It draws techniques from various martial arts, including Judo, Boxing, and Wrestling.
- Defendo training focuses on practical self-defense techniques, situational awareness, and understanding the psychology of confrontations. It emphasizes quick decision-making and adapting to unpredictable situations.
- Defendo incorporates striking, grappling, and weapons defenses, with an emphasis

on simplicity, efficiency, and ending a confrontation as quickly as possible.

These modern self-defense systems offer practitioners practical tools and techniques for real-life self-defense scenarios. They prioritize effectiveness, adaptability, and the ability to neutralize threats quickly. Whether for personal protection, confidence building, or overall physical fitness, these systems provide individuals with practical skills and strategies to navigate potentially dangerous situations.

The role of discipline and respect in martial arts

Discipline and respect are fundamental principles in martial arts, and they play a vital role in the development of practitioners. Here are some key aspects of discipline and respect in martial arts:

1. Self-Discipline:
    - Martial arts cultivate self-discipline, which involves the ability to control one's behavior, emotions, and impulses. Practitioners learn to adhere to training schedules, follow instructions, and maintain a strong work ethic.
    - Self-discipline in martial arts extends beyond the training environment and can positively impact other areas of life, such as academics, work, and personal relationships.

2. Physical Discipline:
    - Martial arts require physical discipline, including regular training, conditioning, and the adherence to proper technique and form. Practitioners develop physical discipline through repetitive practice and the pursuit of continuous improvement.
    - Physical discipline promotes physical fitness, coordination, and overall well-being.

3. Mental Discipline:
    - Martial arts foster mental discipline, which involves focus, concentration, and the ability to remain calm and composed under pressure.

Practitioners learn to control their thoughts and emotions, allowing them to make clear decisions and react appropriately in challenging situations.

- Mental discipline in martial arts extends to the cultivation of resilience, perseverance, and the ability to overcome obstacles.

4. Respect for Instructors and Peers:

- Martial arts instill a deep sense of respect for instructors, trainers, and fellow practitioners. Respect is shown through attentive listening, following instructions, and demonstrating gratitude for the knowledge and guidance received.
- Respect for peers includes treating others with courtesy, fairness, and humility. Practitioners learn to value and appreciate the skills and efforts of others, fostering a supportive and positive training environment.

5. Respect for Tradition and Culture:

- Martial arts often have deep-rooted traditions and cultural significance. Practitioners are encouraged to respect and honor the history, philosophy, and values associated with their chosen art.
- Respect for tradition involves understanding and upholding the principles, etiquette, and customs of the martial art, as well as demonstrating reverence for past masters and their contributions.

Discipline and respect are integral to the martial arts journey. They shape character, instill values, and create an environment conducive to learning and personal growth. Practitioners who embrace discipline and respect develop not only physical prowess but also mental fortitude, humility, and a deep sense of integrity.

The principles of discipline and respect extend beyond the training mat and can positively impact various aspects of life, contributing to personal development, self-improvement, and the fostering of positive relationships within and outside the martial arts community.

The concept of "Do" and its significance

The concept of "Do" is an important aspect of many traditional martial arts and holds significant meaning. Derived from the Japanese term "道" (pronounced "do"), it translates to "the way" or "the path." The concept of "Do" goes beyond physical techniques and encompasses a holistic approach to personal growth and character development. Here are some key aspects of the concept of "Do" and its significance:

1. Character Development:
    - "Do" emphasizes the cultivation of virtues and qualities such as discipline, respect, humility, integrity, and perseverance. Martial arts practitioners strive to embody these principles not only in their training but also in their everyday lives.
    - The pursuit of "Do" encourages practitioners to reflect on their thoughts, actions, and interactions with others, promoting self-improvement and the development of strong character.
2. Mind-Body Connection:
    - "Do" emphasizes the harmonious development of the mind, body, and spirit. Martial arts training is not solely focused on physical techniques but also on mental discipline, focus, and self-awareness.
    - Through training, practitioners learn to control their emotions, develop mental resilience, and cultivate a strong mind-

body connection, allowing them to perform techniques with efficiency and precision.

3. Lifelong Learning:

- The concept of "Do" highlights the idea of continuous learning and improvement. Martial arts practitioners understand that mastery is a lifelong journey and that there is always more to learn and explore.
- Practitioners approach their training with an open mind, remaining receptive to new techniques, insights, and perspectives. They understand that martial arts is a process of constant growth and development.

4. Ethical and Philosophical Foundations:

- "Do" often encompasses ethical and philosophical teachings that guide practitioners' conduct on and off the training mat. It encourages practitioners to embody values such as compassion, honesty, and humility.
- Philosophical teachings associated with "Do" may include concepts such as balance, harmony, and the pursuit of personal enlightenment. These teachings provide a framework for practitioners to navigate challenges and make moral decisions.

5. Application Beyond the Dojo:

- The principles of "Do" extend beyond the confines of the training environment. Practitioners strive to apply the values and lessons learned in martial arts to their everyday lives, relationships, and interactions with others.
- The concept of "Do" encourages practitioners to become positive contributors to their communities, promoting peace, respect, and

personal growth.

In summary, the concept of "Do" represents more than just physical techniques in martial arts. It encompasses a holistic approach to personal growth, character development, and lifelong learning. By embracing the principles of "Do," practitioners strive to cultivate strong character, develop a harmonious mind-body connection, and apply the values learned in martial arts to their daily lives. "Do" serves as a guiding principle that fosters self-improvement, self-discovery, and the pursuit of personal enlightenment.

Cultivating mental and emotional resilience

Cultivating mental and emotional resilience is a crucial aspect of martial arts training. Here are some ways in which martial arts can help develop resilience:

1. Facing Challenges:
    - Martial arts training often presents practitioners with various physical and mental challenges. By regularly pushing their limits and stepping outside their comfort zones, practitioners learn to embrace adversity and develop resilience.
    - Through consistent training, practitioners build mental fortitude, learning to overcome obstacles, handle setbacks, and persevere even when faced with difficulties.

2. Developing a Growth Mindset:
    - Martial arts promote a growth mindset, which is the belief that abilities and skills can be developed through effort and practice. This mindset encourages practitioners to view setbacks and failures as opportunities for learning and growth.
    - By adopting a growth mindset, practitioners cultivate resilience by focusing on continuous improvement, staying motivated, and bouncing back from setbacks with renewed determination.

3. Managing Stress and Pressure:
    - Martial arts training often involves high-

intensity workouts, competitive sparring, and testing situations that simulate real-life confrontations. These experiences help practitioners develop resilience in the face of stress and pressure.

- Through regular exposure to challenging situations, practitioners learn to manage their emotions, stay calm under pressure, and make clear decisions even when faced with intense physical or mental demands.

4. Building Confidence and Self-Efficacy:

- Martial arts training builds confidence and self-efficacy, which contribute to mental and emotional resilience. As practitioners develop their skills, they gain a sense of competence and belief in their ability to handle difficult situations.

- Increased confidence and self-efficacy provide a solid foundation for resilience, as practitioners approach challenges with a positive mindset, believing in their capacity to overcome obstacles and achieve success.

5. Mindfulness and Emotional Regulation:

- Martial arts training often incorporates mindfulness techniques, such as focused breathing and meditation. These practices help practitioners develop self-awareness, emotional regulation, and the ability to stay present in the moment.

- By cultivating mindfulness, practitioners can better manage their emotions, stay focused under pressure, and respond to challenging situations in a calm and controlled manner.

6. Supportive Training Environment:

- Martial arts often foster a supportive and inclusive community. The camaraderie and encouragement from instructors and fellow practitioners provide a valuable support system that enhances resilience.

- The bonds formed in the martial arts community create a sense of belonging, acceptance, and mutual support, which can help practitioners navigate difficult times and bounce back from setbacks.

Cultivating mental and emotional resilience through martial arts is an ongoing process. By consistently facing challenges, adopting a growth mindset, managing stress, building confidence, practicing mindfulness, and benefiting from a supportive training environment, practitioners develop the resilience needed to navigate the physical and mental demands of martial arts training and apply it to their everyday lives.

Harnessing the power of
focus and concentration

Focus and concentration are essential skills in martial arts and can greatly enhance a practitioner's performance. Here are some ways in which martial arts training helps harness the power of focus and concentration:

1. Mind-Body Connection:
   - Martial arts training emphasizes the development of a strong mind-body connection. Through practice, practitioners learn to focus their minds on the present moment, coordinating their thoughts and actions with their physical movements.
   - By training the mind to be fully present, practitioners can improve their focus and concentration, enabling them to execute techniques with precision and efficiency.

2. Attention to Detail:
   - Martial arts require attention to detail, as even small adjustments in technique can have a significant impact on performance. Practitioners learn to concentrate on specific body mechanics, angles, and timing to maximize the effectiveness of their movements.
   - By cultivating attention to detail, practitioners develop a heightened sense of focus, ensuring that every action is deliberate and purposeful.

3. Single-Pointed Focus:
- Martial arts training often involves drills and exercises that require practitioners to focus on a single point or target. Whether it's a specific spot on an opponent's body or a designated area in a training session, practitioners learn to direct their attention and concentrate on that point.
- Single-pointed focus enhances concentration, allowing practitioners to filter out distractions and channel their energy and attention towards their intended target.

4. Mental Discipline:
- Martial arts training fosters mental discipline, which involves the ability to control one's thoughts and maintain focus despite external distractions. Practitioners learn to quiet the mind, block out unnecessary thoughts, and maintain a clear and focused mental state.
- Mental discipline is strengthened through consistent practice and the cultivation of techniques such as meditation and visualization, which help practitioners develop concentration skills and improve their ability to stay focused for extended periods.

5. Pressure Situations:
- Martial arts training exposes practitioners to pressure situations, such as sparring or competitive events. In these situations, the ability to maintain focus and concentration becomes even more crucial.
- Through regular exposure to pressure, practitioners learn to control their emotions, stay composed, and remain focused on the task at hand. This ability to concentrate amidst pressure enhances their overall performance

and decision-making abilities.

6. Mental Training Techniques:
   - Martial arts often incorporate mental training techniques to enhance focus and concentration. These techniques may include visualization exercises, breathing techniques, and mindfulness practices.
   - Visualization involves mentally rehearsing techniques or scenarios, strengthening neural pathways and enhancing concentration. Breathing techniques help regulate the body and mind, promoting relaxation and focus. Mindfulness practices improve self-awareness and present-moment focus.

Harnessing the power of focus and concentration in martial arts requires consistent practice and mental discipline. By cultivating a strong mind-body connection, paying attention to detail, developing single-pointed focus, fostering mental discipline, training under pressure, and utilizing mental training techniques, practitioners can enhance their ability to concentrate and perform at their best in martial arts and in various areas of their lives.

Foundational movements and stances

Foundational movements and stances are fundamental aspects of martial arts training. They provide a solid base from which to execute techniques and contribute to overall balance, stability, and power. Here are some common foundational movements and stances found in martial arts:

1. Horse Stance (Kiba Dachi or Ma Bu):
   - The Horse Stance is a wide-legged stance where the feet are positioned wider than shoulder-width apart, and the knees are bent. The weight is evenly distributed between the legs, and the back is straight.
   - This stance provides stability, lower-body strength, and a strong foundation for generating power in strikes, kicks, and takedowns.
2. Front Stance (Zenkutsu Dachi or Gong Bu):
   - The Front Stance is a long stance where one leg is extended forward with the knee bent and the back leg extended straight. The feet are aligned, and the body weight is distributed mostly on the front leg.
   - This stance emphasizes proper alignment, balance, and forward propulsion, commonly used for delivering powerful strikes and maintaining stability while moving forward.
3. Back Stance (Kokutsu Dachi or Hu Bu):
   - The Back Stance is a stance where one leg is extended back with the knee bent, and the back

leg is straight. The majority of the body weight is on the back leg, and the front foot is turned out slightly.

- This stance provides stability, promotes mobility in multiple directions, and is often used for defensive maneuvers, evasive actions, and generating power for counterattacks.

4. Cat Stance (Neko Ashi Dachi or Mao Bu):

- The Cat Stance is a short, narrow stance where one foot is placed beside the other foot, with the knees slightly bent. The body weight is primarily on the back leg.
- This stance is used for quick transitions, balance, and agility. It allows practitioners to swiftly change direction, evade attacks, and set up counterattacks.

5. Fighting Stance or Guard Position:

- The Fighting Stance, also known as the Guard Position, is a balanced stance used for combat. The feet are shoulder-width apart, knees are slightly bent, and the body is angled slightly sideways.
- This stance provides mobility, balance, and readiness to defend and attack. It allows practitioners to move quickly in any direction and protects vulnerable areas of the body.

In addition to these stances, martial arts also incorporate various foundational movements, such as stepping, pivoting, lunging, and shifting weight. These movements enhance footwork, agility, and overall body coordination.

Practicing and mastering foundational movements and stances is essential for building a strong martial arts foundation. They serve as the building blocks for executing techniques with power, precision, and efficiency. Through consistent practice and attention to detail, practitioners develop the necessary body mechanics, balance, and stability to progress in their martial arts journey.

Striking techniques and combinations

Striking techniques and combinations are integral parts of martial arts training. They involve the effective use of punches, kicks, elbows, and knees to strike an opponent. Here are some common striking techniques and combinations used in various martial arts disciplines:

1. Jab:
   - The jab is a quick and straight punch thrown with the lead hand. It is used to set up other strikes, maintain distance, and probe an opponent's defenses.

2. Cross:
   - The cross is a powerful punch thrown with the rear hand, usually following a jab. It involves rotation of the hips and shoulders, generating significant power. It is often aimed at the opponent's head or body.

3. Hook:
   - The hook is a curved punch thrown with a bent arm, targeting the opponent's head or body from the side. It is effective in close-range fighting and can generate significant power.

4. Uppercut:
   - The uppercut is an upward punch thrown from a lower angle, usually targeting the opponent's chin or body. It is effective at close range and can be used to surprise an opponent by coming up from underneath their guard.

5. Roundhouse Kick:

- The roundhouse kick is a powerful kick delivered by swinging the leg in a circular motion. The kick is typically aimed at the opponent's body or head, using the shin or instep as the striking surface.

6. Front Kick:

- The front kick is a straight kick delivered with the ball of the foot or the heel. It is typically aimed at the opponent's midsection, providing both offense and defense by creating distance.

7. Side Kick:

- The side kick involves extending the leg sideways and striking the opponent with the heel or outer edge of the foot. It is effective for pushing an opponent away or striking their midsection.

8. Elbow Strike:

- Elbow strikes involve using the elbow as a striking weapon. Various elbow strikes, such as the horizontal elbow, downward elbow, and spinning elbow, can be used in close-quarters combat.

9. Knee Strike:

- Knee strikes involve driving the knee into an opponent's body, usually targeting the midsection, thighs, or head. They are powerful strikes used at close range or in clinching situations.

10. Combinations:

- Combinations involve linking together multiple strikes in quick succession to create effective and unpredictable attacks. For example, a common combination may be a jab-cross-hook or a roundhouse kick followed by a cross.

Remember, proper technique, body mechanics, and timing are crucial for executing striking techniques effectively. It is essential to practice under the guidance of a qualified instructor and focus on developing speed, accuracy, and power while maintaining control. Regular training and repetition will help refine striking techniques and combinations, enabling practitioners to apply them efficiently in self-defense or competitive situations.

Grappling techniques and submissions

Grappling techniques and submissions are fundamental aspects of martial arts that focus on close-range combat, controlling an opponent, and submitting them through joint locks or chokes. Here are some common grappling techniques and submissions used in various martial arts disciplines:

1. takedowns:
   - Takedowns involve techniques used to bring an opponent from a standing position to the ground. Examples include single-leg takedowns, double-leg takedowns, and hip throws. Takedowns are often used to establish control and initiate ground grappling.

2. Mount:
   - The mount is a dominant position where the person on top straddles the opponent's torso, placing their legs on either side. From the mount, the practitioner can strike, transition to submissions, or control the opponent's movements.

3. Side Control:
   - Side control is a position where the practitioner is on top of the opponent, perpendicular to their body, with their chest pressing against the opponent's side. It offers control over the opponent's upper body, allowing for submissions and transitions to other positions.

4. Guard:
   - The guard is a defensive position where the

practitioner is on their back, using their legs and hips to control the opponent. From the guard, various sweeps, submissions, and attacks can be launched.

5. Rear Naked Choke:

- The rear naked choke is a submission that involves applying pressure to the opponent's neck from the rear. It is executed by wrapping an arm around the opponent's neck, securing a grip, and applying pressure with the forearm.

6. Armbar:

- The armbar is a submission that targets the opponent's arm joint, typically the elbow. It involves controlling the opponent's arm, extending it, and applying pressure to hyperextend the joint.

7. Triangle Choke:

- The triangle choke is a submission that involves trapping the opponent's head and arm between the practitioner's legs, creating a triangular shape. Pressure is applied by squeezing the legs together and manipulating the opponent's posture.

8. Kimura Lock:

- The Kimura lock targets the opponent's shoulder joint. It involves securing the opponent's arm, manipulating it into an unnatural position, and applying pressure to force a submission or create a positional advantage.

9. Guillotine Choke:

- The guillotine choke is a submission that targets the opponent's neck. It involves wrapping an arm around the opponent's neck, securing a grip, and applying pressure by squeezing the arm and body together.

10. Rear Naked Choke:

- The rear naked choke is a highly effective submission that targets the opponent's neck from the rear. It involves wrapping an arm around the opponent's neck, securing a grip, and applying pressure with the forearm to cut off blood flow to the brain.

It is important to note that grappling techniques and submissions can vary depending on the martial art style and ruleset. Training in grappling arts such as Brazilian Jiu-Jitsu, Judo, or wrestling can provide a deeper understanding of these techniques and how to effectively apply them in both self-defense situations and competitive settings. Proper technique, control, and respect for the safety of training partners are crucial when practicing grappling techniques and submissions.

Forms, katas, and patterns

Forms, katas, and patterns are predetermined sequences of movements and techniques practiced in martial arts. They serve as a training tool for developing various aspects of martial arts, including technique, balance, coordination, timing, and focus. Here is an overview of forms, katas, and patterns in different martial arts disciplines:

1. Forms (also known as "Poomsae" or "Hyung"):
   - Forms are practiced in disciplines such as Taekwondo, Karate, and Kung Fu. They consist of a series of movements, strikes, kicks, and defensive techniques performed in a specific order and pattern.
   - Forms help practitioners develop muscle memory, proper technique, and fluidity of movement. They often include elements of self-defense scenarios and traditional philosophies.

2. Katas:
   - Katas are practiced in disciplines such as Karate, Judo, and Kung Fu. They are choreographed patterns of movements and techniques performed against imaginary opponents.
   - Katas emphasize precision, focus, and the application of techniques in a controlled manner. They help practitioners develop proper body alignment, breathing, and mental discipline.

3. Patterns (also known as "Poomsae" or "Tul"):

- Patterns are practiced in disciplines such as Taekwondo and Hapkido. They consist of a set sequence of movements, including strikes, kicks, and blocks, performed with fluidity and precision.
- Patterns provide a structured way to practice techniques, footwork, and stances while promoting balance, coordination, and concentration. They often have a deeper meaning and represent specific principles or concepts within the martial art.

4. Forms in Kung Fu:

- Kung Fu incorporates various forms that can be categorized into external styles (such as Shaolin Kung Fu) and internal styles (such as Tai Chi). These forms focus on developing physical strength, flexibility, and martial skill while incorporating elements of philosophy and self-discipline.

5. Forms in Japanese Martial Arts:

- Japanese martial arts like Karate, Aikido, and Judo have specific forms or katas associated with their respective styles. These forms aim to refine technique, cultivate a focused mindset, and preserve the traditional aspects of the martial art.

The practice of forms, katas, and patterns varies across martial arts styles and schools. They are typically learned and performed individually or in groups, with practitioners aiming to execute each movement with precision, fluidity, and control. Regular practice of forms, katas, and patterns helps develop muscle memory, improve technique, deepen understanding of martial arts principles, and enhance overall performance in self-defense or competitive situations.

Sparring and competition training

Sparring and competition training are essential components of many martial arts disciplines. They provide practitioners with opportunities to apply their skills in a dynamic and controlled environment, test their abilities against opponents, and develop important attributes such as timing, distance management, and strategy. Here is an overview of sparring and competition training in martial arts:

1. Sparring:
   - Sparring is a form of practice or training that involves simulated combat with an opponent. It allows practitioners to apply their techniques, strategies, and defensive skills in a dynamic and interactive setting.
   - Sparring can be practiced in various formats, ranging from light contact or controlled sparring to full-contact sparring, depending on the martial arts style, school, and personal goals.
   - It helps develop attributes such as timing, accuracy, speed, reflexes, and adaptability. It also enhances situational awareness, decision-making, and the ability to execute techniques under pressure.

2. Competitive Training:
   - Competitive training focuses on preparing practitioners for martial arts competitions, tournaments, or matches. It involves specific training strategies and drills aimed at

developing skills and attributes required for successful competition.

- Competitive training may include practicing specific techniques, refining strategies, conditioning exercises, mental preparation, and simulated competition scenarios.
- It helps practitioners develop the ability to perform under pressure, handle the intensity of a competitive environment, and adapt to different opponents and rule sets.

3. Rules and Safety:

- In both sparring and competitive training, adherence to specific rules and safety guidelines is crucial. These rules are designed to ensure the safety of the participants and maintain a fair and controlled environment.
- Rules may vary depending on the martial arts style and the level of competition. They often dictate the allowed target areas, prohibited techniques, equipment requirements, and scoring criteria.
- Safety measures, such as the use of protective gear (e.g., mouthguards, helmets, gloves) and appropriate supervision, are implemented to minimize the risk of injuries during sparring or competition.

4. Benefits of Sparring and Competition Training:

- Sparring and competition training offer several benefits to martial arts practitioners, including:
  - Improved reflexes, timing, and coordination.
  - Enhanced physical conditioning and endurance.
  - Increased self-confidence and mental resilience.

- Better understanding of practical application of techniques.
- Opportunity to assess and refine one's skills and abilities.
- Exposure to different styles and approaches through interactions with opponents.
- Development of sportsmanship, respect, and humility.

It is important to note that sparring and competition training should be conducted under the guidance of qualified instructors, with an emphasis on safety and proper technique. Practitioners should gradually progress from controlled and supervised training to more intense or competitive environments as they develop their skills and gain experience.

Profiles of influential martial artists throughout history

Throughout history, there have been numerous influential martial artists who have made significant contributions to the development and popularization of martial arts. Here are profiles of some of these influential figures:

1. Bodhidharma (5th/6th century):
    - Bodhidharma, also known as Daruma in Japan, is credited with bringing the teachings of Zen Buddhism to China and the Shaolin Temple. He is believed to have developed a system of physical exercises and meditation known as "Yijin Jing," which laid the foundation for the martial arts practiced at the Shaolin Temple.

2. Miyamoto Musashi (1584-1645):
    - Miyamoto Musashi was a renowned Japanese swordsman and strategist. He is best known for his book "The Book of Five Rings," which offers insights into strategy, tactics, and the martial arts mindset. Musashi's approach to combat, known as "Niten Ichi-ryu," emphasized the use of both a sword and a shorter companion weapon simultaneously.

3. Yip Man (1893-1972):
    - Yip Man was a Chinese martial artist and the primary teacher of the Wing Chun style of Kung Fu. He is most famous for being the teacher of Bruce Lee. Yip Man played a crucial

role in preserving and spreading Wing Chun, which became one of the most popular and influential martial arts styles in the world.

4. Helio Gracie (1913-2009):

- Helio Gracie was a Brazilian martial artist and one of the founders of the martial art of Brazilian Jiu-Jitsu (BJJ). He developed a modified version of Japanese Jiu-Jitsu, which emphasized leverage, technique, and ground fighting. Gracie's efforts popularized BJJ and revolutionized the world of martial arts, particularly in the realm of ground combat and mixed martial arts (MMA).

5. Bruce Lee (1940-1973):

- Bruce Lee was a Chinese-American martial artist, actor, and philosopher. He is considered a cultural icon and one of the most influential martial artists of all time. Bruce Lee's approach to martial arts, known as Jeet Kune Do, emphasized simplicity, practicality, and adaptability. His philosophy and innovative training methods had a profound impact on martial arts, film, and popular culture.

6. Mas Oyama (1923-1994):

- Mas Oyama, also known as Choi Yeong-eui, was a Korean-Japanese martial artist who founded Kyokushin Karate. He is renowned for his incredible physical and mental strength, as well as his emphasis on rigorous training and full-contact sparring. Oyama's Kyokushin Karate is characterized by its focus on discipline, physical conditioning, and strong striking techniques.

7. Zhang Sanfeng (12th/13th century):

- Zhang Sanfeng is a legendary figure in Chinese martial arts and is often considered the creator of Tai Chi Chuan. Legend has it that Zhang Sanfeng was an accomplished martial artist and Daoist philosopher who developed Tai Chi based on principles of balance, internal energy cultivation, and harmonizing with the opponent's force.

These are just a few examples of influential martial artists throughout history. Each of them has left a lasting impact on the development and evolution of martial arts, both in their respective regions and globally. Their contributions in terms of philosophy, techniques, and training methods continue to inspire and shape the practice of martial arts today.

Their philosophies, contributions, and legacies

1. **Bodhidharma:**
   - **Philosophy:** Bodhidharma's teachings blended Zen Buddhism with physical training, emphasizing the integration of mind and body.
   - **Contributions:** He is credited with developing the physical exercises and meditation practices that laid the foundation for the martial arts practiced at the Shaolin Temple.
   - **Legacy:** Bodhidharma's influence can be seen in the Shaolin martial arts, which incorporate physical conditioning, meditation, and a focus on the mind-body connection.

2. **Miyamoto Musashi:**
   - **Philosophy:** Musashi's philosophy emphasized the importance of mastering oneself, achieving spiritual enlightenment, and adopting a flexible approach to combat and life.
   - **Contributions:** Musashi's book, "The Book of Five Rings," has become a classic text on strategy, influencing martial artists and businessmen alike. His approach to swordsmanship and strategy continues to shape the practice of martial arts.
   - **Legacy:** Musashi's teachings on strategy, mental focus, and adaptability have had a lasting impact not only on martial arts but also on various fields, including business, leadership, and personal development.

3. **Yip Man:**

- Philosophy: Yip Man emphasized the principles of efficiency, economy of motion, and simultaneous attack and defense in Wing Chun. He also highlighted the importance of cultivating a humble and disciplined mindset.
- Contributions: Yip Man's teaching played a crucial role in preserving and spreading the Wing Chun style, which has become one of the most popular and influential martial arts in the world. His students, including Bruce Lee, further propagated the style.
- Legacy: Yip Man's legacy lies in the continued practice and evolution of Wing Chun, which has had a significant influence on the development of martial arts, particularly in the realm of close-quarters combat.

4. Helio Gracie:

- Philosophy: Gracie's philosophy emphasized leverage, technique, and the concept that a smaller, weaker person can overcome a larger opponent through skill and strategy.
- Contributions: Helio Gracie's development of Brazilian Jiu-Jitsu (BJJ) revolutionized ground fighting and had a profound impact on mixed martial arts (MMA). He popularized BJJ and established the Gracie family as prominent figures in the martial arts world.
- Legacy: Gracie's legacy is the ongoing global practice and evolution of BJJ. It continues to be a cornerstone of MMA and self-defense systems, and the Gracie family remains highly respected in the martial arts community.

5. Bruce Lee:

- Philosophy: Bruce Lee's philosophy emphasized the importance of adaptability, self-expression, and personal growth. He advocated for a holistic approach to martial arts and encouraged practitioners to develop their own unique style.

- Contributions: Bruce Lee's innovative training methods, philosophy, and approach to combat through Jeet Kune Do had a profound influence on the martial arts world. He popularized martial arts in the mainstream and inspired countless practitioners.
- Legacy: Bruce Lee's legacy lies in his impact on martial arts philosophy, his contributions to film and popular culture, and his role in promoting the idea of martial arts as a path of self-discovery and personal development.

6. Mas Oyama:

- Philosophy: Oyama's philosophy centered around discipline, perseverance, and the pursuit of physical and mental strength. He believed in the transformative power of rigorous training and full-contact sparring.
- Contributions: Mas Oyama founded Kyokushin Karate, which emphasized physical conditioning, strong striking techniques, and full-contact sparring. He popularized the concept of breaking objects to demonstrate martial arts prowess.
- Legacy: Oyama's legacy is the global practice of Kyokushin Karate and its influence on other martial arts. His emphasis on physical conditioning, discipline, and full-contact training has had a significant impact on martial arts training methods and competitive fighting.

These influential martial artists have left lasting legacies through their philosophies, contributions, and teachings. Their ideas and techniques continue to inspire practitioners worldwide, shaping the way martial arts are practiced, taught, and understood.

Lessons we can learn from their experiences

The experiences of influential martial artists offer valuable lessons that can be applied not only to martial arts training but also to various aspects of life. Here are some lessons we can learn from their experiences:

1. Embrace discipline and perseverance: Martial arts require discipline and consistent practice. The dedication and perseverance shown by these influential martial artists serve as a reminder of the importance of commitment and hard work in achieving success in any endeavor.

2. Cultivate a growth mindset: Many of these martial artists emphasized the importance of continuous learning and self-improvement. They encourage us to adopt a growth mindset, where we view challenges as opportunities for growth and approach each practice session or obstacle with a desire to learn and improve.

3. Emphasize the integration of mind and body: The teachings of these martial artists highlight the connection between the mind and body. They remind us of the importance of cultivating mental resilience, focus, and self-awareness, as well as developing physical strength, coordination, and agility.

4. Adaptability and flexibility: Bruce Lee, in particular, emphasized the importance of being adaptable and open to different approaches. The ability to adjust and adapt to changing circumstances is a valuable skill not only in martial arts but also in life.

5. Embrace the journey and enjoy the process: The martial

arts journeys of these influential figures teach us to appreciate the process of learning and self-discovery. They remind us that mastery is a lifelong pursuit and that the real value lies in the journey itself, rather than just the destination.

6. Cultivate humility and respect: Respect for oneself and others is a core value in martial arts. The examples set by these martial artists remind us of the importance of humility, respect, and sportsmanship in our interactions with others, both on and off the training mat.

7. Apply martial arts principles beyond the training room: The philosophies and principles espoused by these martial artists can be applied to various aspects of life. Whether it is the strategic thinking of Miyamoto Musashi, the adaptability of Bruce Lee, or the discipline of Mas Oyama, their teachings can help us navigate challenges, set goals, and find balance in our personal and professional lives.

These lessons serve as valuable guidance for practitioners of martial arts and anyone seeking personal growth and development. By incorporating these lessons into our lives, we can not only improve our martial arts skills but also cultivate a mindset and approach that can lead to success and fulfillment in various areas.

Mental and emotional benefits of martial arts training

Martial arts training offers numerous mental and emotional benefits that can positively impact overall well-being. Here are some of the mental and emotional benefits of practicing martial arts:

1. Improved focus and concentration: Martial arts training requires mental focus and concentration. Through techniques such as meditation, forms, and sparring, practitioners learn to sharpen their attention, block out distractions, and focus on the present moment. This enhanced focus can carry over into other areas of life, improving productivity and performance.

2. Increased self-confidence: Martial arts training builds self-confidence by providing practitioners with a sense of accomplishment as they progress in their skills and overcome challenges. The knowledge of self-defense techniques and the ability to protect oneself can boost self-esteem and instill a sense of empowerment.

3. Stress relief and emotional well-being: Engaging in physical activity releases endorphins, which are natural mood-boosting chemicals in the brain. Regular martial arts training can help reduce stress, anxiety, and depression, promoting overall emotional well-being. The structured nature of martial arts classes also provides a healthy outlet for emotional expression and stress management.

4. Enhanced self-discipline and self-control: Martial

arts training instills discipline and self-control as practitioners adhere to the rules and principles of their chosen style. The practice of techniques, adherence to a training schedule, and following the guidance of instructors promote self-discipline, helping individuals develop the ability to control their impulses and make healthier choices.

5. Improved resilience and mental toughness: Martial arts training challenges practitioners both physically and mentally, pushing them out of their comfort zones. This process helps develop resilience and mental toughness, as individuals learn to push through obstacles, handle setbacks, and persist in the face of adversity. These skills can be applied to other areas of life, such as work, relationships, and personal goals.

6. Increased self-awareness and emotional intelligence: Martial arts training encourages self-reflection and introspection, promoting self-awareness. Through practice, individuals learn to better understand their own strengths, weaknesses, and emotions. This heightened self-awareness can lead to improved emotional intelligence, better interpersonal relationships, and more effective communication skills.

7. Mind-body connection: Martial arts training emphasizes the integration of mind and body, teaching practitioners to be present and aware of their body's movements and sensations. This mind-body connection enhances body awareness and coordination, while also promoting a sense of harmony and balance between physical and mental well-being.

It is important to note that the mental and emotional benefits of martial arts training may vary for each individual, and the experience can be influenced by the specific style, instructor, and training environment. However, overall, martial arts training provides a holistic approach to physical and mental well-being, fostering personal growth and development.

Building self-confidence and self-awareness

Building self-confidence and self-awareness are important aspects of martial arts training. Here's how practicing martial arts can help develop these qualities:

1. Skill mastery: As individuals progress in their martial arts training, they acquire new skills and techniques. Mastering these skills, such as strikes, kicks, or grappling moves, helps build self-confidence as practitioners see their progress and feel more capable in their abilities.
2. Overcoming challenges: Martial arts training often presents physical and mental challenges that require perseverance and resilience. As practitioners face and overcome these challenges, they develop a sense of accomplishment and confidence in their ability to handle difficult situations.
3. Positive reinforcement: Instructors and training partners provide feedback and encouragement, reinforcing progress and achievements. This positive reinforcement helps individuals build confidence in their abilities and fosters a positive self-image.
4. Self-defense knowledge: Learning self-defense techniques provides individuals with a sense of security and empowerment. Knowing that they can protect themselves in dangerous situations boosts self-confidence and enhances overall self-awareness.
5. Self-reflection and introspection: Martial arts training encourages self-reflection and introspection. Through techniques like forms, meditation, and mindfulness

exercises, practitioners develop a deeper understanding of themselves. This self-reflection helps build self-awareness and improves the ability to regulate emotions and respond effectively in different situations.

6. Embracing strengths and weaknesses: Martial arts training highlights both strengths and weaknesses. It helps individuals recognize their natural abilities and areas for improvement. By acknowledging and working on weaknesses, individuals build self-awareness and develop strategies for growth and self-improvement.

7. Constructive feedback: Instructors and training partners provide constructive feedback during training sessions. This feedback helps individuals gain insight into their performance and areas where they can improve. Accepting and integrating this feedback fosters self-awareness and a willingness to grow and learn.

8. Mind-body connection: Martial arts training emphasizes the integration of mind and body. Through practicing techniques, individuals develop a deeper awareness of their body's movements, capabilities, and limitations. This increased mind-body connection enhances self-awareness and promotes a sense of self-confidence and control.

By engaging in regular martial arts training, individuals can build self-confidence and self-awareness, leading to a positive self-image and a greater understanding of themselves. These qualities can be applied not only in martial arts but also in various aspects of life, helping individuals navigate challenges, make confident decisions, and cultivate a strong sense of self.

Stress relief and mental well-being

Martial arts training offers significant benefits for stress relief and overall mental well-being. Here's how practicing martial arts can help alleviate stress and promote mental well-being:

1. Physical activity and endorphin release: Engaging in martial arts training involves physical activity, which releases endorphins in the brain. Endorphins are natural chemicals that act as mood elevators and promote feelings of well-being and happiness. Regular physical activity through martial arts can reduce stress, anxiety, and depression.

2. Focus and mindfulness: Martial arts training requires mental focus and concentration. When practicing techniques or sparring, practitioners need to be fully present in the moment, concentrating on their movements and the task at hand. This focus on the present moment helps shift attention away from stressors, promoting mindfulness and reducing anxiety.

3. Stress management techniques: Martial arts often incorporate stress management techniques, such as breathing exercises, meditation, and visualization. These techniques help individuals calm their minds, relax their bodies, and reduce the impact of stress on their overall well-being.

4. Outlet for frustration and tension: Martial arts training provides a safe and structured outlet for releasing frustration, tension, and pent-up energy. Striking pads or engaging in controlled sparring allows individuals to physically express their emotions and release built-up

stress and tension in a controlled environment.

5. Increased self-confidence: Martial arts training builds self-confidence as individuals progress in their skills and achieve goals. This increased self-confidence helps individuals better manage stress by fostering a positive self-image, enhancing problem-solving abilities, and promoting resilience in the face of challenges.

6. Social support and camaraderie: Martial arts training often takes place in a supportive and inclusive community. The camaraderie and support from training partners and instructors can alleviate feelings of isolation and provide a sense of belonging. The social aspect of martial arts can enhance mental well-being by fostering connections, promoting positive relationships, and providing emotional support.

7. Emotional regulation and self-control: Martial arts training emphasizes discipline and self-control. Through practice, individuals learn to regulate their emotions, manage impulses, and respond to challenging situations with composure. This enhanced emotional regulation promotes mental well-being and helps individuals cope with stress in a healthier and more balanced way.

8. Sense of achievement and purpose: Setting goals and working towards achieving them in martial arts training provides a sense of purpose and accomplishment. The sense of achievement gained from progressing in skills and overcoming challenges can boost self-esteem, improve motivation, and contribute to overall mental well-being.

By engaging in regular martial arts training, individuals can experience stress relief, improved mental well-being, and a greater sense of balance in their lives. The combination of physical activity, focus, stress management techniques, social support, and personal growth contributes to an overall sense of calm, resilience, and mental well-being.

Balancing physical and mental development

Balancing physical and mental development is a fundamental aspect of martial arts training. Here are some key considerations for achieving this balance:

1. Holistic Approach: Martial arts training is not solely focused on physical fitness and techniques. It also emphasizes mental and emotional growth. By recognizing and embracing the holistic nature of martial arts, practitioners can strive for a balanced development of their mind and body.

2. Mindfulness and Focus: Martial arts training encourages practitioners to cultivate mindfulness and focus. Through techniques like meditation, breathing exercises, and visualization, individuals can develop mental clarity, enhance concentration, and improve their ability to be fully present in the training session.

3. Mental Resilience: Martial arts training challenges individuals both physically and mentally. It pushes practitioners to their limits, helping them develop mental resilience and the ability to overcome obstacles. Techniques such as sparring and competition provide opportunities to test mental strength, adaptability, and problem-solving skills.

4. Incorporating Mental Training: Alongside physical conditioning, martial arts training can include specific mental training exercises. These may involve visualization techniques, mental rehearsal of techniques, and developing strategies for handling stress and pressure. Integrating mental training into

regular practice sessions helps develop a well-rounded approach to martial arts.

5. Self-Reflection and Self-Awareness: Martial arts training encourages self-reflection and self-awareness. Practitioners are encouraged to assess their strengths, weaknesses, and areas for improvement. This introspective process allows individuals to identify mental patterns, emotional responses, and thought processes that may influence their performance and personal growth.

6. Positive Mindset and Growth Mindset: Martial arts training promotes a positive mindset and a growth mindset. Practitioners learn to embrace challenges, view setbacks as opportunities for growth, and believe in their ability to improve. By adopting a growth mindset, individuals can approach both physical and mental challenges with resilience, determination, and a willingness to learn.

7. Rest and Recovery: Balancing physical and mental development requires adequate rest and recovery. Overtraining or neglecting rest can lead to physical injuries, mental burnout, and diminished performance. Practitioners should prioritize quality sleep, incorporate rest days into their training schedule, and engage in activities that promote relaxation and stress reduction.

8. Guidance from Instructors: Instructors play a crucial role in helping practitioners strike a balance between physical and mental development. They provide guidance, mentorship, and feedback to ensure that training programs address both aspects. Instructors can also provide resources and support for mental training techniques and facilitate discussions on mental well-being.

By consciously integrating physical and mental development into martial arts training, practitioners can experience holistic growth, improved performance, and a greater sense of well-being. This balance not only enhances martial arts skills but also extends to other areas of life, fostering resilience, self-awareness, and personal growth.

Martial arts in warfare and self-defense throughout history

Martial arts have played a significant role in warfare and self-defense throughout history. Here's an overview of their historical importance in these contexts:

1. Martial Arts in Warfare:
    - Ancient Civilizations: Martial arts techniques were developed and practiced by ancient civilizations such as China, Japan, Greece, and India. These techniques were used in warfare to train soldiers in hand-to-hand combat, weapon usage, and battlefield strategies.
    - Historical Martial Arts: Various martial arts systems were specifically developed for warfare. For example, in Japan, the samurai class developed the martial art of kenjutsu (swordsmanship), while in Europe, knights and soldiers trained in fencing and wrestling techniques.
    - Military Combat Systems: Many military organizations and special forces around the world incorporate martial arts training into their programs. These systems, such as Krav Maga used by the Israeli Defense Forces, focus on practical and efficient self-defense techniques suitable for real-life combat situations.
2. Martial Arts for Self-Defense:

- Traditional Martial Arts: Martial arts systems like Karate, Taekwondo, and Jiu-Jitsu originated as self-defense arts, with techniques designed to enable individuals to protect themselves from physical threats.
- Street Self-Defense: Over time, various martial arts styles adapted their training methodologies to address self-defense needs in modern urban environments. Systems like Krav Maga, Systema, and Jeet Kune Do emphasize practical techniques for real-world self-defense scenarios.
- Women's Self-Defense: Martial arts training has been embraced by women as a means of self-defense, empowerment, and personal safety. Many martial arts schools now offer specialized programs and techniques tailored for women's self-defense needs.
- Martial Arts for Personal Safety: Martial arts training provides individuals with the skills, confidence, and awareness necessary to protect themselves and others from potential dangers. The focus on situational awareness, physical techniques, and mental preparedness equips practitioners with the tools to navigate potentially threatening situations.

Throughout history, martial arts have evolved and adapted to meet the changing needs of warfare and self-defense. While their applications may vary, the underlying principles of discipline, technique, and strategy remain fundamental. Martial arts training continues to serve as a means for individuals to protect themselves, develop physical and mental strength, and cultivate a sense of personal security and confidence.

Influence of martial arts on popular culture and media

Martial arts have had a profound influence on popular culture and media, shaping various forms of entertainment and leaving a lasting impact. Here are some ways in which martial arts have influenced popular culture:

1. Martial Arts Films: Martial arts films, especially those from Hong Kong and East Asia, have gained international popularity. Films featuring iconic martial artists like Bruce Lee, Jackie Chan, Jet Li, and Donnie Yen have captivated audiences with their impressive fighting skills, choreography, and storytelling. These films have introduced martial arts to a global audience and inspired countless individuals to pursue martial arts training.

2. Martial Arts in Action Movies: Martial arts techniques and styles have become integral components of action movies across different genres. From Hollywood blockbusters to international cinema, fight scenes featuring martial arts have become synonymous with excitement and high-energy action. Martial arts choreographers and performers contribute their skills to create visually stunning and dynamic fight sequences.

3. Martial Arts Video Games: Martial arts have influenced the world of video games, with many games featuring characters skilled in various martial arts styles. Games like Street Fighter, Tekken, Mortal Kombat, and Virtua

Fighter have incorporated martial arts moves and techniques into their gameplay, allowing players to engage in virtual combat using a wide range of martial arts-inspired fighting styles.

4. Mixed Martial Arts (MMA): The rise of MMA, with organizations like the Ultimate Fighting Championship (UFC), has brought martial arts into the mainstream sports world. MMA combines techniques from various martial arts disciplines, including striking, grappling, and submission holds. The popularity of MMA has led to increased interest in martial arts training and a broader understanding of different styles.

5. Martial Arts Television Series: Martial arts themes and storylines are featured in numerous television series, both in live-action and animated formats. Shows like Kung Fu, Avatar: The Last Airbender, and Dragon Ball have showcased martial arts skills, philosophies, and moral lessons, influencing audiences and sparking an interest in martial arts.

6. Martial Arts Fashion and Iconography: Martial arts attire, such as the traditional gis (uniforms), belts, and martial arts-themed clothing, have become fashionable in popular culture. Martial arts symbols and icons, such as the yin and yang, dragon, and tiger, are widely recognized and incorporated into fashion, accessories, and merchandise.

7. Martial Arts as Fitness and Wellness: Martial arts-inspired fitness programs, like kickboxing and cardio martial arts, have gained popularity as effective workouts that combine martial arts techniques with cardiovascular exercises. These programs attract individuals who seek a fun and engaging way to stay fit and improve their overall well-being.

The influence of martial arts on popular culture and media has not only introduced martial arts to wider audiences but also helped shape the perception of martial arts as a disciplined art form, a physical activity, and a source of inspiration. The portrayal of martial arts in entertainment has motivated individuals to explore martial arts training, leading to increased participation and appreciation for the discipline.

Martial arts tournaments and their impact

Martial arts tournaments have a significant impact on practitioners, spectators, and the martial arts community as a whole. Here are some ways in which martial arts tournaments influence and contribute to the martial arts world:

1. Competitive Spirit and Skill Development: Tournaments provide a platform for martial artists to showcase their skills, test their abilities, and compete against other practitioners. The competitive atmosphere fosters a sense of determination, pushing participants to improve their techniques, physical fitness, and mental focus. Tournaments often serve as a driving force for practitioners to train harder, refine their skills, and reach new levels of proficiency.

2. Community Building: Tournaments bring martial artists together from various styles, schools, and backgrounds. Participants have the opportunity to meet and interact with fellow practitioners, forging connections and building a sense of camaraderie within the martial arts community. This fosters a supportive and collaborative environment where practitioners can learn from one another, exchange knowledge, and develop friendships that extend beyond the tournament experience.

3. Exposure and Recognition: Martial arts tournaments provide a platform for talented practitioners to gain exposure and recognition for their skills. Exceptional performances in tournaments can lead to opportunities for sponsorship, media coverage, and invitations to

participate in prestigious events. This recognition not only validates the hard work and dedication of the practitioners but also raises the profile of their martial arts style and school.

4. Skill Evaluation and Feedback: Tournaments offer an objective evaluation of a practitioner's skills and progress. Competing against other skilled individuals allows practitioners to gauge their abilities and identify areas for improvement. Feedback from judges and coaches helps participants gain insights into their strengths and weaknesses, enabling them to focus their training efforts and continue their development.

5. Personal Growth and Character Development: Participating in tournaments requires discipline, perseverance, and mental fortitude. The preparation, nerves, and challenges faced during competition contribute to personal growth and character development. Practitioners learn to manage stress, overcome setbacks, and display good sportsmanship, cultivating valuable life skills that extend beyond the tournament arena.

6. Inspiration and Motivation: Witnessing high-level performances and displays of skill at tournaments can be a powerful source of inspiration and motivation for both participants and spectators. Spectators, especially aspiring martial artists, are often inspired by the dedication, passion, and technical prowess demonstrated by tournament competitors. This inspiration fuels their own martial arts journey, encouraging them to set goals, train diligently, and strive for excellence.

7. Promotion of Martial Arts Styles: Tournaments showcase the diversity of martial arts styles, allowing practitioners and spectators to witness the unique characteristics and techniques of various disciplines. This exposure helps promote different martial arts

styles and raises awareness about their history, philosophy, and cultural significance.

Martial arts tournaments serve as important milestones in the martial arts journey, offering opportunities for growth, recognition, and connection within the martial arts community. They inspire practitioners to push their limits, foster a sense of unity, and contribute to the overall development and progression of martial arts as a whole.

Choosing the right martial art for you

Choosing the right martial art is a personal decision that depends on your individual preferences, goals, and circumstances. Here are some factors to consider when selecting a martial art:

1. Purpose and Goals: Determine why you want to practice martial arts. Are you interested in self-defense, physical fitness, competition, stress relief, or personal development? Clarifying your purpose and goals will help narrow down the options.

2. Martial Arts Styles: Research different martial arts styles and their philosophies, techniques, and training methodologies. Each style has its unique focus, such as striking (e.g., Karate, Muay Thai), grappling (e.g., Brazilian Jiu-Jitsu, Judo), or a combination of both (e.g., MMA). Consider which style aligns with your interests and goals.

3. Instructor and School: The quality of instruction and the atmosphere of the school are crucial factors in your martial arts journey. Visit different schools, observe classes, and speak with instructors and students to assess their teaching style, experience, and values. Ensure that the school's culture and values align with your own.

4. Accessibility and Schedule: Consider the location of the school and the schedule of classes. Choose a martial art that is accessible to you, whether it's near your home, workplace, or school. Additionally, consider whether the class schedule fits into your lifestyle and availability.

5. Physical Requirements: Take into account your current

fitness level, flexibility, and any existing injuries or physical limitations. Some martial arts may be more physically demanding than others, so choose a style that suits your physical capabilities and allows for gradual progression.

6. Personal Preferences: Consider your personal preferences in terms of training environment, class structure, and learning format. Some people enjoy the formality and structure of traditional martial arts, while others prefer a more relaxed and informal atmosphere. Decide what type of environment will motivate and inspire you to consistently train.

7. Trial Classes: Many martial arts schools offer trial classes or introductory packages. Take advantage of these opportunities to experience the training firsthand. Participating in a class will help you gauge your comfort level, the teaching style, and whether it's a good fit for you.

8. Long-Term Commitment: Martial arts require dedication and long-term commitment to see progress and reap the benefits. Consider whether you are ready to invest time, effort, and resources into training consistently.

Remember that the journey of martial arts is ongoing, and your preferences and goals may evolve over time. It's okay to try different martial arts styles and schools until you find the right fit for you. The most important factor is to choose a martial art that resonates with you and brings you joy and fulfillment in your practice.

Finding the right instructor and training environment

Finding the right instructor and training environment is crucial for a positive and fulfilling martial arts experience. Here are some factors to consider when evaluating instructors and training environments:

1. Qualifications and Experience: Look for instructors who have relevant qualifications, certifications, and extensive experience in their martial art. They should have a solid understanding of the techniques, principles, and philosophy of the martial art they teach. Consider their rank, training lineage, and any notable accomplishments in their martial arts journey.

2. Teaching Style and Approach: Every instructor has their own teaching style and approach. Some instructors may focus more on technique and precision, while others prioritize practical application and real-world scenarios. Observe classes or participate in trial sessions to get a sense of the instructor's teaching methods and how well they resonate with your learning style.

3. Communication and Instruction: Effective communication is essential for a productive learning experience. A good instructor should be able to explain techniques clearly, provide constructive feedback, and answer students' questions. They should also create a supportive and inclusive learning environment where students feel comfortable asking for help and clarification.

4. Emphasis on Safety and Injury Prevention: Safety should be a top priority in any martial arts training environment. Instructors should enforce proper safety protocols, such as warm-ups, stretching, and appropriate use of protective gear. They should also emphasize the importance of proper technique and discourage reckless or unsafe behavior during training.

5. Class Structure and Curriculum: Consider the structure and organization of the classes. Are they well-planned, progressive, and catered to the needs of different skill levels? A good instructor will have a structured curriculum that allows for systematic learning and development, ensuring that students are continually challenged and making progress.

6. Student Progression and Support: An instructor should be invested in their students' progress and development. They should provide opportunities for students to test and advance in rank, such as belt promotions or grading exams. Additionally, a supportive instructor will offer guidance and support outside of class, helping students set goals and providing resources to aid in their progression.

7. Training Atmosphere and Culture: The training environment and the culture of the school play a significant role in your overall experience. Pay attention to the atmosphere during classes. Is there a positive and respectful atmosphere where students support and encourage one another? Consider whether the school's values align with your own and if you feel comfortable and welcomed within the community.

8. Reputation and Reviews: Seek recommendations from other martial artists, friends, or online communities. Read reviews and testimonials about the instructor and the school to gather insights from current and past students. While individual experiences may vary, this can provide some guidance in your decision-making

process.

Remember, finding the right instructor and training environment may require some exploration and trial classes. Trust your instincts and choose an instructor and school that resonate with you, provide quality instruction, and foster a supportive and inclusive learning environment.

Setting goals and tracking progress

Setting goals and tracking progress is essential for maintaining motivation and measuring your growth in martial arts. Here are some tips for setting goals and effectively tracking your progress:

1. Define Clear and Specific Goals: Set clear, specific, and realistic goals that align with your martial arts aspirations. Whether it's earning a certain belt rank, mastering a particular technique, or competing in a tournament, clarity in your goals will help guide your training and provide a sense of direction.

2. Break Down Goals into Milestones: Break down your larger goals into smaller, achievable milestones. This allows you to track progress more effectively and provides a sense of accomplishment as you reach each milestone. For example, if your goal is to compete in a tournament, your milestones could include regular sparring sessions, refining specific techniques, and improving conditioning.

3. Use SMART Goals: Apply the SMART goal-setting framework to make your goals more effective. SMART stands for Specific, Measurable, Achievable, Relevant, and Time-bound. Ensure that your goals are specific, quantifiable, attainable, relevant to your martial arts journey, and have a specific timeline attached to them.

4. Keep a Training Journal: Maintain a training journal or logbook to document your training sessions, progress, and reflections. Record details such as techniques learned, training drills, sparring experiences, and personal observations. This journal serves as a

valuable tool for tracking progress, identifying areas for improvement rank, and reflecting on your martial arts journey.

5. Regularly Assess and Evaluate: Regularly assess your progress to evaluate your development and identify areas for improvement. This can be done through self-reflection, feedback from instructors or training partners, or participating in periodic belt tests or evaluations. Honest self-assessment helps you stay focused, adjust your training as needed, and set new goals.

6. Seek Feedback and Guidance: Actively seek feedback and guidance from your instructor, training partners, and more experienced martial artists. They can provide valuable insights, corrections, and advice that contribute to your growth. Be open to constructive criticism and use it as an opportunity to refine your techniques and skills.

7. Celebrate Achievements: Celebrate your accomplishments along the way. Whether it's mastering a new technique, winning a sparring match, or earning a higher belt rank, acknowledging and celebrating your achievements boosts motivation and reinforces your progress.

8. Adapt and Adjust Goals as Needed: As you progress in your martial arts journey, you may need to adapt and adjust your goals. This can be due to changing interests, new aspirations, or unforeseen circumstances. Be flexible and willing to revise your goals to ensure they continue to align with your evolving martial arts path.

Remember that progress in martial arts is a journey, and improvement takes time and consistent effort. By setting clear goals, tracking your progress, and staying committed to your training, you can continue to grow and evolve as a martial artist.

Overcoming challenges and staying motivated

Overcoming challenges and staying motivated in martial arts can be a rewarding yet demanding task. Here are some strategies to help you navigate obstacles and maintain motivation:

1. Embrace the Learning Process: Recognize that challenges and setbacks are an integral part of the martial arts journey. Instead of viewing them as failures, see them as opportunities for growth and learning. Embrace the process of improvement, understanding that progress takes time and consistent effort.

2. Set Realistic Expectations: Avoid setting overly lofty or unrealistic expectations for yourself. Martial arts mastery is a lifelong pursuit, and progress comes in increments. Set achievable goals and celebrate small victories along the way to stay motivated and maintain a positive mindset.

3. Find Your Why: Reflect on your reasons for practicing martial arts. Identify the deeper motivations and personal benefits that drive you. Whether it's self-defense, personal growth, physical fitness, or stress relief, connecting with your "why" can provide a source of inspiration during challenging times.

4. Break Down Big Goals: If you have long-term goals, break them down into smaller, manageable steps. This helps prevent overwhelm and allows you to focus on making progress one step at a time. Celebrating achievements at each milestone boosts motivation and reinforces your commitment.

5. Surround Yourself with Supportive People: Seek out a supportive community of fellow martial artists, instructors, and training partners who uplift and encourage you. Surrounding yourself with like-minded individuals who share your passion for martial arts can provide valuable support, guidance, and motivation.

6. Mix Up Your Training: Avoid falling into a rut by diversifying your training routine. Explore different training methods, attend seminars or workshops, try new techniques, or cross-train in complementary disciplines. Variety keeps training fresh and exciting, preventing boredom and boosting motivation.

7. Visualize Success: Use visualization techniques to envision yourself achieving your martial arts goals. Visualize yourself executing techniques flawlessly, overcoming challenges, and succeeding in your endeavors. This mental imagery can help boost confidence and motivation, as your mind begins to believe in your capabilities.

8. Find Inspiration: Seek inspiration from martial arts movies, books, documentaries, or interviews with accomplished martial artists. Hearing about others' journeys, learning from their experiences, and witnessing their dedication can reignite your passion and provide a fresh perspective.

9. Take Breaks and Rest: It's important to listen to your body and give yourself adequate rest and recovery. Overtraining can lead to burnout and diminishing motivation. Allow yourself time to rest, rejuvenate, and recharge, so you can come back to training with renewed energy and enthusiasm.

10. Keep a Positive Mindset: Cultivate a positive mindset by focusing on progress rather than perfection. Celebrate your achievements, no matter how small, and maintain a sense of gratitude for the opportunity to train in martial arts. Surround yourself with positive

affirmations and maintain an optimistic outlook, even during challenging times.

Remember that motivation may fluctuate, and it's natural to encounter obstacles along your martial arts journey. By implementing these strategies and staying committed to your training, you can overcome challenges, maintain motivation, and continue to grow as a martial artist.

Reflection on the transformative power of martial arts

The transformative power of martial arts is undeniable. It goes far beyond physical fitness and self-defense skills, permeating into various aspects of life. Here are some reflections on the transformative power of martial arts:

1. Self-Confidence and Empowerment: Martial arts instill a deep sense of self-confidence and empowerment. As you learn and master techniques, overcome challenges, and achieve personal milestones, your confidence grows. This newfound confidence extends beyond the martial arts mat and positively influences how you carry yourself in everyday life.

2. Discipline and Focus: Martial arts require discipline and focus, teaching practitioners to set goals, follow training schedules, and maintain consistent practice. Through this discipline, you develop the ability to focus your mind, block out distractions, and concentrate on the task at hand. These skills can be applied to other areas of life, such as work, academics, and personal relationships.

3. Mental Resilience: Martial arts training builds mental resilience by pushing you beyond your comfort zone and challenging your limits. You learn to embrace discomfort, persevere through difficult situations, and develop a "never give up" attitude. These mental skills enable you to navigate life's challenges with greater resilience and determination.

4. Emotional Regulation: Martial arts provide an outlet for emotional expression and help develop emotional regulation skills. Through training, you learn to channel your emotions effectively, manage stress, and control aggression. This emotional intelligence can lead to healthier relationships, better decision-making, and improved overall well-being.

5. Conflict Resolution and Peaceful Mindset: Martial arts emphasize non-violent conflict resolution and promote a peaceful mindset. Contrary to popular belief, martial artists strive to avoid confrontation whenever possible and prioritize harmony and respect. This mindset extends to daily interactions, fostering a greater sense of empathy, understanding, and peaceful coexistence.

6. Mind-Body Connection: Martial arts emphasize the integration of the mind and body. Through training, you develop body awareness, coordination, and control. This mind-body connection enhances overall physical performance, balance, and agility. Moreover, it promotes mindfulness, as you learn to be present in the moment and attuned to the sensations of your body.

7. Character Development: Martial arts place great emphasis on character development, nurturing qualities such as integrity, humility, perseverance, and respect. The principles and values instilled in martial arts training can positively influence your behavior, relationships, and moral compass.

8. Community and Camaraderie: Martial arts provide a supportive and inclusive community of like-minded individuals who share a passion for personal growth and self-improvement. The camaraderie within martial arts communities fosters a sense of belonging and support, offering a network of individuals who inspire and uplift one another.

9. Lifelong Learning: Martial arts are a lifelong journey of learning and growth. There is always something

new to discover, techniques to refine, and challenges to overcome. The commitment to continuous learning cultivates a growth mindset, encourages curiosity, and fuels personal development throughout all stages of life.

10. Personal Transformation: Perhaps the most profound aspect of martial arts is the potential for personal transformation. As you embark on this journey, you may discover hidden strengths, break through self-imposed limitations, and tap into a deeper sense of purpose and self-awareness. Martial arts can shape not only your physical capabilities but also your character, mindset, and outlook on life.

In conclusion, the transformative power of martial arts extends beyond physical prowess. It touches the mind, spirit, and character, fostering personal growth, self-confidence, discipline, resilience, and a peaceful mindset. The journey through martial arts is a lifelong pursuit that continually shapes and transforms individuals, empowering them to become the best version of themselves both inside and outside the training space.

Final thoughts and encouragement for readers

In closing, I would like to offer some final thoughts and encouragement to readers on their martial arts journey:

1. Embrace the Journey: Martial arts is a lifelong journey filled with ups and downs. Embrace every step along the way, both the triumphs and the challenges. Each experience contributes to your growth and development as a martial artist and as an individual.

2. Stay Committed: Consistency is key in martial arts. Make a commitment to your training and prioritize it in your life. Even when motivation wavers, remember your passion and the benefits that martial arts bring to your life.

3. Embrace Growth Mindset: Approach martial arts with a growth mindset. Embrace the process of learning, be open to feedback and correction, and view setbacks as opportunities for improvement. Embrace the idea that there is always more to learn and room for growth.

4. Support and Encourage Others: Martial arts is not just an individual pursuit, but also a community. Support and encourage your training partners and fellow martial artists. Share your knowledge, offer a helping hand, and celebrate their successes. Together, you can create a positive and empowering environment.

5. Seek Balance: Find balance between your martial arts training and other aspects of your life. Prioritize self-care, maintain healthy relationships, and pursue other interests outside of martial arts. A balanced approach will contribute to your overall well-being and longevity

in the martial arts journey.

6. Enjoy the Process: Remember to enjoy the process of training and the joy of movement. Martial arts can be physically demanding, but it is also a source of inspiration, joy, and personal expression. Find moments of fun and gratitude in each training session.

7. Believe in Yourself: Believe in your abilities and potential as a martial artist. Trust that you have what it takes to overcome challenges and reach your goals. Self-belief and a positive mindset are powerful allies in your martial arts journey.

8. Never Stop Learning: Martial arts is a vast and ever-evolving discipline. Never stop learning and exploring new techniques, styles, and philosophies. Seek out opportunities for growth, attend seminars, workshops, and continue to expand your knowledge and skillset.

9. Celebrate Your Progress: Take the time to celebrate your achievements, both big and small. Each step forward is a testament to your dedication and hard work. Acknowledge and appreciate your progress, as it fuels motivation and confidence.

10. Remember Why You Started: During challenging times, reflect on the reasons why you started your martial arts journey. Reconnect with the passion, purpose, and personal benefits that drew you to martial arts in the first place. Let those reasons be a source of inspiration and a reminder of the transformative power of martial arts.

In the pursuit of martial arts, remember that it is not just about achieving belts or mastering techniques—it is a path of personal growth, self-discovery, and empowerment. Stay committed, stay curious, and embrace the transformative journey that lies ahead. Keep pushing your boundaries, believing in yourself, and always strive to unleash the warrior within.

Best wishes on your martial arts journey!

Resources for further exploration

If you're interested in further exploring the world of martial arts, here are some resources that can be helpful:

1. Books: There are numerous books available on various martial arts disciplines, their history, philosophy, techniques, and more. Some recommended titles include "The Tao of Jeet Kune Do" by Bruce Lee, "The Book of Five Rings" by Miyamoto Musashi, "Aikido and the Dynamic Sphere" by Adele Westbrook and Oscar Ratti, and "Jiu-Jitsu University" by Saulo Ribeiro.

2. Online Courses and Video Tutorials: Many martial arts instructors and organizations offer online courses and video tutorials that can help you deepen your understanding of specific styles and techniques. Platforms such as Udemy, YouTube, and specialized martial arts websites often have a wealth of instructional content available.

3. Martial Arts Websites and Forums: Explore martial arts websites and forums to find articles, discussions, and resources related to your specific interests. Websites such as Black Belt Magazine, Martial Arts Planet, and Reddit's r/martialarts community are great places to connect with fellow enthusiasts and gain insights from experienced practitioners.

4. Martial Arts Schools and Instructors: Consider finding a reputable martial arts school or instructor in your area. Direct instruction and guidance from qualified instructors can enhance your learning experience and provide valuable feedback and support. Research

different schools, read reviews, and visit them in person to find the right fit for you.

5. Martial Arts Documentaries and Films: Documentaries and films can provide an immersive and entertaining way to learn about martial arts history, culture, and the journeys of influential practitioners. Some noteworthy documentaries include "The Last Samurai" (2003), "The Karate Kid" (1984), "The Warrior's Way" (2010), and "Enter the Dragon" (1973).

6. Martial Arts Events and Seminars: Attend martial arts events, seminars, and workshops to expand your knowledge, learn from experts, and connect with the broader martial arts community. These events often feature demonstrations, training sessions, and opportunities for networking and further exploration.

7. Martial Arts Magazines: Subscribe to martial arts magazines such as Black Belt Magazine, Kung Fu Tai Chi Magazine, or Martial Arts Illustrated. These publications often feature interviews, articles, training tips, and insights from renowned martial artists.

8. Historical and Cultural Studies: Delve into the historical and cultural aspects of martial arts by exploring books, academic papers, and documentaries that shed light on the origins, development, and cultural significance of various martial arts styles.

Remember, while these resources can provide valuable information and inspiration, hands-on training under the guidance of a qualified instructor is essential for proper technique, safety, and progression in martial arts. Enjoy your exploration of martial arts, and may it bring you a deeper understanding and appreciation for this rich and diverse discipline!